CW00547473

A Geezer's Guide to

MULLET MAINTENANCE AND COMBOVER CARE

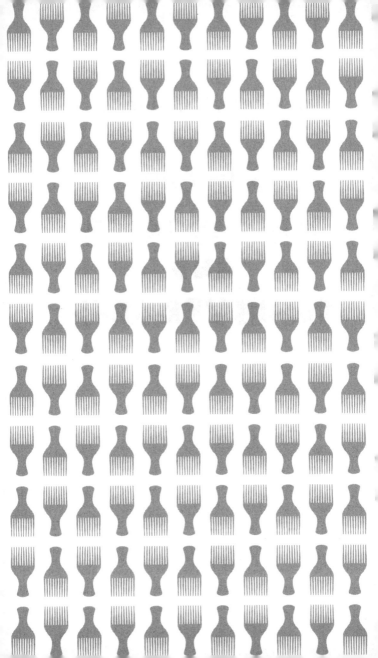

A Geezer's Guide to

MULLET MAINTENANCE AND COMBOVER CARE

Chris Martin

The History Press

front cover illustration: © istockphoto

First published 2013

The History Press
The Mill, Brimscombe Port
Stroud, Gloucestershire, GL5 2QG
www.thehistorypress.co.uk

© Chris Martin, 2013

British Library Cataloguing in Publication Data.
A catalogue record for this book is available from the British Library.

ISBN 978 0 7524 8921 6

Typesetting and origination by The History Press
Printed in Great Britain
Manufacturing managed by Jellyfish Solutions Ltd

Contents

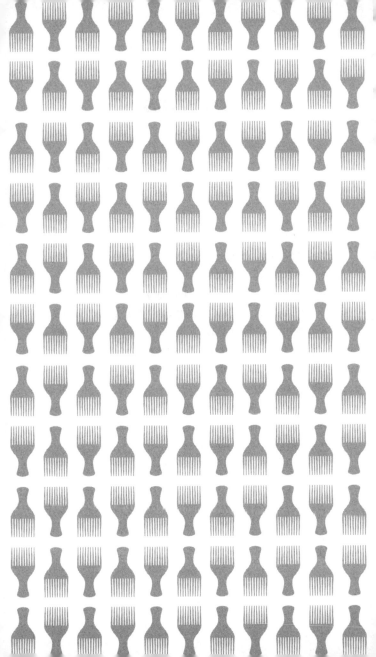

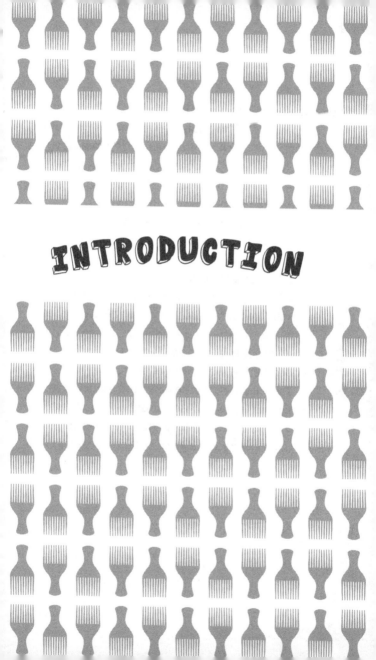

INTRODUCTION

It was the thirteenth-century cleric William of Wykeham who first argued, 'manners maketh the man'. Such a sentiment may have flown in medieval times, but the modern geezer on the go is aware that – nowadays – there is a little more to it than remembering your Ps and Qs.

By what yardstick does our fast-moving society judge a man? Is it his car, his mobile phone or his watch? No. Is it his ability to run a marathon maybe, or give CPR, or change a spark plug? Surely not. In our fashion-conscious world, it is his haircut that sets a man apart, for better or worse. While some say we should judge a man solely on the contents of his head, most of us are more concerned by what he's got on it.

This may seem a little harsh, but modern men no longer have any excuse for debuting a disastrous 'do. At no time in history have they had access to such an incredible range of potential styles, as well as the state-of-the-art technologies and styling aids to ensure their barnets look the business.

In this book, we will tell you all you need to know about making your mullet magnificent. We'll trace the history of the man mop from the Mongols to Metrosexuals, taking in some of the world's most famous manes along the way. There are tips on hair care and hairstyling, and even some terrible warnings from the salon chair brought to vivid life by the very worst of celebrity follicle-focused meltdowns.

Our aim is to demonstrate that a decent trim is not just something you need for a job interview, a first date or a wedding, but the gateway to a whole new life of confidence and charisma. A real geezer knows that a good hairstyle says more about you than a million column inches ever could, so whether you choose a DA or Dreadhawk, a parting or a ponytail, this book can help you make sure your 'do is always the dog's ...

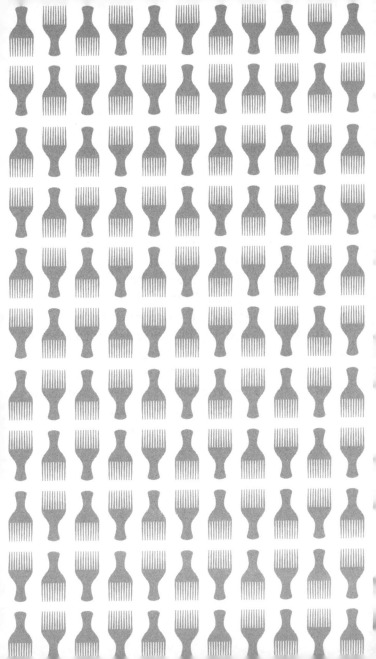

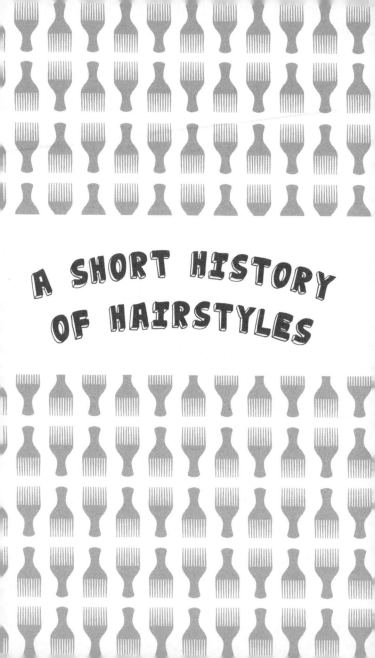

A SHORT HISTORY OF HAIRSTYLES

You only need to look at the story of Samson and Delilah to see just how important a man's hairstyle can be. In this epic Bible story the famously strong man was stripped of his powers by the loss of his locks. While this cautionary tale has inspired writers, sculptors, composers and screenwriters throughout the ages, Samson's drape is just one of a long list of classic men's hairstyles over the centuries. What follows is a whistle-stop journey through the hairdos that shaped the world of men as we know it.

Ancient World

Having just evolved from apes and with the first professional hairdresser still several centuries away, it is safe to assume that primeval man must have rocked some kind of Shag cut, even though it may have been difficult to distinguish it from the rest of his abundant body hair. As early and primitive societies formed, the first formal hairstyles began to evolve, with men's long unruly hair being tied back with hide bands. However, men soon evolved further to use iron or bronze shears to crudely crop their unruly bangs in an effort to control it. By the time of the Babylonian and Assyrian Empires, men were going further than just cropping and began to deliberately style their hair, growing it long and dyeing it black, as well as creating crimping and curling effects with hot irons to set off their long square beards.

The Ancient Egyptians chose to wear their hair very short and even shaved their heads to deal with the desert heat. Sexually ambiguous members of the royal elite would cover their bald domes with elaborate headdresses and wigs held in place with beeswax and resin. These were cut into short symmetrical shapes or styled into long braids before being adorned with ivory hairpins, flowers or golden ornaments. But by the time of the Golden Age of Greece such gender-bending flamboyance was gone, as the Greeks – with their focus on logic and reason – favoured short, pragmatic haircuts.

Roman Empire

Probably the most famous do of the Roman era was created by the emperor Julius Caesar who wore his hair short, brushed forward from the crown and oiled flat against his scalp. Though the Imperial trim set off a laurel crown delightfully, such Caesar cuts had not always been popular in Ancient Rome. In the early – more austere – days of the Republic, Roman men generally followed simple styles inspired by their Greek forebears. It was in the later years of Imperial Rome that the Romans' narcissism (helped by the fact that they ruled most of the known world) ushered in a whole new age.

Barbering had been introduced to Rome from the Greek colonies of Sicily in 296 BC. Though public barbers were originally used by those who could not afford to keep a slave to cut their hair, the new shops quickly became popular as a venue to catch up on local gossip and political moves in the Senate. As a bonus, these first barbers doubled up as surgeons and dentists, so as well as a haircut and shave, they'd throw in blood-letting, cupping, leeching and even the odd enema. Access to these new (relatively) skilled hairstylists, combined with the wild extravagance of the times, saw the upper classes fashioning elaborate ringlets with curling irons and dusting their hair with coloured powders or – for those committed to the kind of super bling that would put P Diddy to shame – gold dust.

Middle Ages

Following the collapse of the Roman Empire, the Germanic barbarians who overran Europe preferred to focus more on destruction and mayhem than hairdressing. They favoured long, flowing (unwashed) locks and straggly beards – a bit like a nation of psychotic Gandalfs. One ruling family of the barbarian era, the Merovingians, were often referred to as the 'long-haired kings' (Latin *reges criniti*) as their unchecked hair growth clearly distinguished them from the more civilised Franks, who commonly cut their hair short. These barbarians attached great importance to their hair. How long a man's hair was became a symbol of power and authority, and in battle they tied their tresses in a high Top Knot to appear taller and more terrifying to their short-haired enemies. Indeed, outside of being caught flipping through interior-decoration magazines with his knitting circle, the worst humiliation a barbarian could face was to lose his hair; as a result slaves and war prisoners were routinely shorn to complete their humiliation.

Near the end of the tenth century, the Catholic Church, seeking to curtail the power of the barbarian kings, began to issue edicts against the length of men's hair. Excommunication by Rome meant the loss of a king's authority to rule, so these edicts meant Christian kings had to get a haircut and shave pronto or risk being unseated. The results saw a movement towards shoulder-length hair. This was often neatly rolled at the neck to create the Page Boy style, or for the less fashion conscious (e.g. peasants), cut crudely into a Pudding-basin. The clergy were distinguished in society by the Tonsure, a deeply unflattering shaved patch on the top of the head, designed to mimic Christ's crown of thorns.

Renaissance

The Renaissance was a time of philosophical and cultural revolution across Europe, ushering a new era of scientific endeavour. It also led to a change in hairstyles as freethinkers harked back once more to Ancient Greece and begin to cut their locks off. Legend has it that this trend was further accelerated when Francis I of France accidentally burned off his hair with a torch and his subjects cut their hair shorter in sympathy – usually combining it with a fruity little beard and moustache combo.

But as time went on, men inevitably yearned once again for flamboyance. Hair began to grow longer as dedicated followers of fashion wore long, curled tresses, often oiled and falling over wide, white collars. This style was sometimes accessorised with a single longer lock hanging down the back, tied with a velvet bow.

Super camp monarchism came face to face with stone-face Puritanism during the English Civil War, and such fey beautification understandably became a symbol of division between the warring sides. Followers of Oliver Cromwell decided to crop their hair close to their head as an act of defiance towards the curls and ringlets of the king's men. This led to the Parliamentary faction's New Model Army having better-fitting helmets and to be nicknamed 'Roundheads'.

Louis XIV and the Rise of the Wig

Across the Channel, France was still some years from a revolution of their own and men had no such qualms about going completely poodle with their dos. With the growth of poorly sanitised, plague-ridden cities leaping with nits, it was perhaps inevitable that men would choose to crop their locks and turn to wigs to achieve the bubble perms they craved. Without the requirement to be able to grow their own hair, the shape, styling and sheer size of the wig became a sign of status in seventeenth-century France. King Louis XIV – the Sun King – led the way with his truly extravagant and mind-bogglingly expensive horse-hair constructions. For the next two centuries men adopted wigs as their preferred look, creating a new source of income for designers and manufacturers of such hair pieces. The first wig makers' guild was established in France in 1665. It was a development that was soon copied elsewhere in Europe as the new industry of making, rather than styling hair, flourished.

Regency Era

In the eighteenth century, men's wigs became smaller and more formal, usually an arrangement of strict partings and tight-rolled curls. Men of the day also took to powdering their wigs to give their syrups a distinctive white colour. Increasingly the style of wig a man wore was associated with his profession, with the law, the army, and the navy each having their own style of wig.

But all that powdering and wig care was an expensive and messy business, so by the end of the century, young blades including the soon-to-be American President, George Washington, were simply curling and powdering their own hair to see if anyone noticed the difference. They didn't.

In 1795, the British Government levied a tax on hair powder of 1 guinea per year. This tax effectively caused the end of the wearing of both wigs and powder, as tight-fisted Brits chose to go *au naturelle* rather than fork out for fashion. By the 1780s the move away from wigs was complete. The reaction against such formality and its associated costs led to the Hérisson (hedgehog) style being adopted; a return to a loose, bushy mass of curls.

It is worth noting that hairdressers – as opposed to barbers – now began to form a distinct profession for the first time. Ironically many of this new breed of hairsmiths had originally trained as wig makers. Most notable was Legros de Rumigny, who became court hairdresser in France and opened an *Academie de Coiffure* in 1769 to promote the art of hairdressing.

Victorian Era

Freed from the tyranny of powdering their head several times a day, and generally more concerned with commerce, converting baffled natives to Christianity and building gigantic things out of iron, Victorian men spent less time on their hair. Throughout the nineteenth century they kept it relatively short, sometimes curled and usually dressed with macassar oil. Just as in previous austere times, men sought to balance the paucity of opportunity for expression on the top of their heads with a variety of moustaches, sideburns and monstrous spade beards; the author Charles Dickens should receive special credit, both for his contribution to literature and his remarkable Combover.

Twentieth Century

Men's hair in the early part of the twentieth century was generally simple and short. Well-dressed men wore well-groomed styles which were trimmed close to flatter the shape of the head, neatly parted and usually held in place with a generous dollop of Brilliantine. Such styles were created in the newly established men's hairdressing salons that offered a choice of scissor or razor cuts, plus an array of oils and tonics. The Crew Cut was also formalised in this period, when the rowing team at Yale had their hair cut short in an effort to distinguish themselves from members of the university's football team, who wore their hair (relatively) long for extra padding under their leather helmets. Severe haircuts persisted throughout the 1920s, '30s and '40s, not least due to the fact that many men were drafted to serve in the armed forces during the First and Second World Wars.

However, in the 1950s a new kind of rebellious youth culture began to assert itself. Rock 'n' roll icons like James Dean and Elvis Presley made pompadour hairstyles such as the Ducktail popular among wannabe bad boys. Indeed Elvis' hair was so revered that thousands of his fans staged public protests when the US Army cut off the King's hair during his military service. But it was in the 1960s that youth culture really went into overdrive, as nonconformist young men tuned in, turned on and grew their hair long. These new anti-'dos did more than merely compliment a snazzy set of psychedelic clothes; long hair became the cornerstone of the hippie revolution. In short, the rejection of the values inherited from previous generations was expressed through the medium of hair. In 1967 this sentiment was embodied in the first rock opera – simply called *Hair*.

By the 1970s almost every level of society had adapted their dress and hairstyles to reflect the new liberalism, resulting in Shag Cuts, Feather Cuts, early proto-Mullets and some frankly ill-advised bell-bottom trousers.

Thankfully during the 1980s there was a spring back towards more restrained styles as the new 'yuppies' (young urban professionals) chose more conservative business cuts, focusing instead on size and volume enhanced by blow drying and the generous application of gel or mousse.

Nowadays pretty much anything goes. Advanced hairdressing techniques mean dyeing, curling, straightening and styling are easier than ever before. The result is that there has never been more diversity in the hairstyles worn by all generations. Walk down the street in any large city and you'll see Bowl Cuts and Dreadlocks right next to Quiffs and Bubble perms, as each man makes an individual choice based on personal style, rather than the dictates of society.

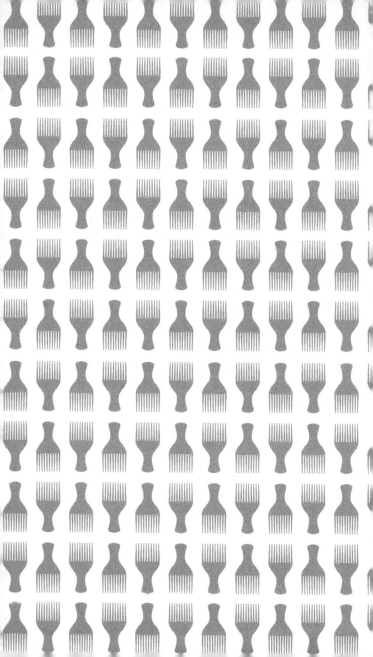

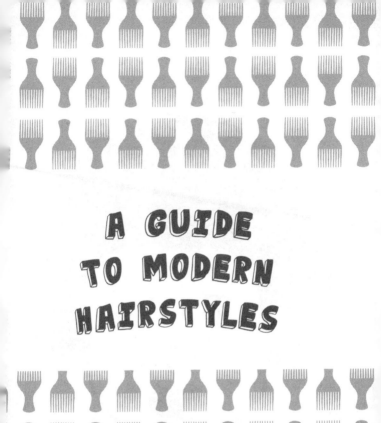

A GUIDE
TO MODERN
HAIRSTYLES

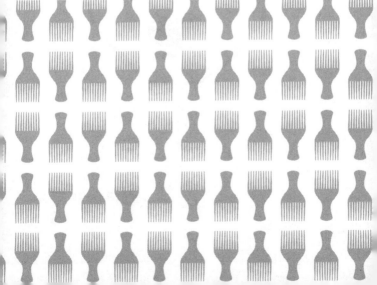

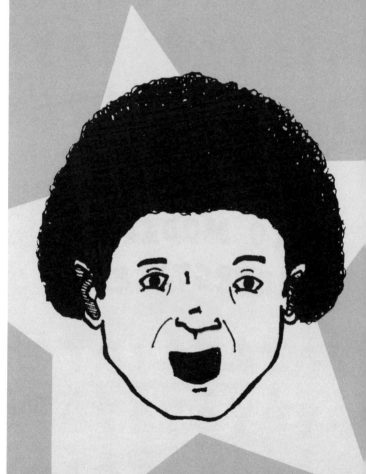

COOL
RATING

AFRO

Think flares. Think medallions. Think purple furs and gold-rimmed glasses. Think chequerboard dance floors that spell a one-night ticket to boogie wonderland. The Afro went from being the preserve of mad scientists and meths-drinking tramps to the height of sophistication during the disco boom of the 1970s. Sometimes shortened to a 'Fro and also known as a Natural, you will need long kinky or curly hair as well as platform boots and a pocket full of 'ludes to pull this off. The hairstyle is created by simply combing the hair away from the scalp, allowing it to extend out from the head in a large, rounded shape, much like a funky halo bestowed by the gods of getting down. This style is usually seen on people of colour but the good news is there's nothing to stop anyone from becoming an undercover brother if they've been blessed with a natural frizz. Then the style is better known as a Jewfro.

✂ Try to look like **Lenny Kravitz**
✂ Try not to look like **Phil Spector**

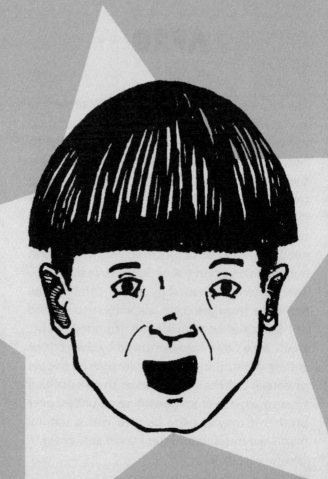

COOL
RATING

BOWL CUT

Synonymous with children leaping with nits, medieval foot soldiers and members of punk band The Ramones, the Bowl Cut is a cheap and easy option for people who don't want to try too hard. Also known as a Pot Cut, Helmet Cut or Mushroom Cut, the Bowl Cut is fashioned by allowing the hair to fall naturally from the crown of the head before cutting it along a horizontal line around the sides and back, to create the impression that someone put a bowl on your head and trimmed your hair around it. It takes its name both from its distinct shape and from the traditional method of creating it (i.e. literally putting a bowl on a person's head). The cut's striking symmetry and unashamed simplicity will appeal to you if you see your head garden as part fashion statement, part practical head gear and part return to childhood, which probably accounts for its recent resurgence among dungaree-wearing, dummy-sucking fans of the rave scene.

✂ Try to look like **Ian Brown** from The Stone Roses
✂ Try not to look like **Moe Howard** from The Three Stooges

A GUIDE TO MODERN HAIRSTYLES

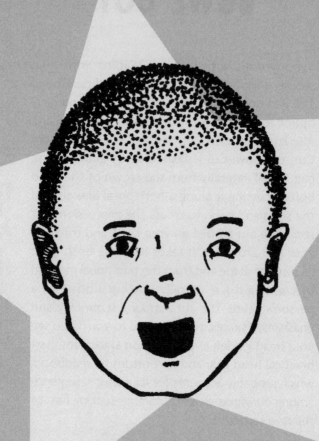

COOL
RATING

BUZZ CUT

Popular with red necks, ex-military drill sergeants, macho lesbians and working-class children on the first day of a new school term, the Buzz Cut is a no-nonsense, no-style tribute to masculine hairdressing, that tells the world you're both pragmatic and the chances are that you've recently received an ASBO. A Buzz Cut describes any style where the hair is cut aggressively close to the head with electric clippers so that no more than three-quarters of an inch of growth remains on all sides. Also known as the Butch Cut and the Crew Cut, this trim was originally used to stop the spread of lice. It's worth considering a Buzz Cut if you can't afford a decent haircut, or you can't be bothered to decide what haircut you want, or if you just fancy looking like you've been recently featured on *Crimewatch*. There is one other way to end up with a Buzz Cut: forget to tip your stylist.

✂ Try to look like **Justin Timberlake**
✂ Try not to look like **P!nk**

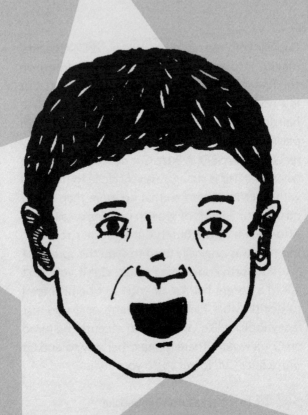

COOL
RATING

CAESAR CUT

Modelled on an ancient bust of Emperor Julius Caesar, the Caesar Cut is a heavily styled creation which harks back to the glorious days of the Roman Empire. The hair is cut short and brushed forward horizontally towards the face before being greased down. Favoured by confused teens, poets and people who have recently suffered a nervous breakdown, the Caesar Cut is a triumph of the use of products over skilful hairdressing, as well as a fast track to an acne-speckled forehead. While you may feel this 'do is reminiscent of marching legions, three-day orgies and brutal gladiatorial action, unless you're over 6ft and built like a brick bathhouse, you'll look more like a Hobbit from *Lord of the Rings*.

✂ Try to look like **Maximus Decimus Meridius**, Commander of the Armies of the North, General of the Felix Legions, loyal servant to the true emperor, Marcus Aurelius

✂ Try not to look like **Frodo Baggins**

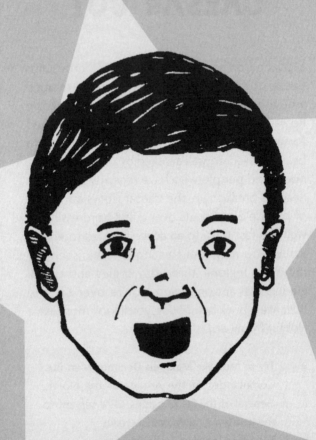

COOL
RATING

CLASSIC TAPER

If you work nine to five in a stuffy, open-plan office, wear a suit and spend your day looking at spreadsheets, the chances are you're a business man and you have a Classic Taper on you head. Sometimes referred to as a Business Man's Cut or a Graduation, the Classic Taper is a very traditional men's trim that is appropriate for any lifestyle that involves eating lunch at Pret a Manger five days a week. The hair is cut with a slight taper on the sides and back, and the top is left long enough to part and comb to the side. It is smart, easy to maintain and enduringly popular among working professionals who require a conservative look. Over the course of this century the Classic Taper has been long and short, greased close to the head, buffed and glossed by Brylcreem, moussed, even blow dried into something resembling a bird's wing, but at its heart, the same simple, parted style, remains. Much like apple pie, Coca Cola and the photocopier in your office, if it ain't broke, don't fix it.

✄ Try to look like **John Hamm**
✄ Try not to look like **Crispin Glover**

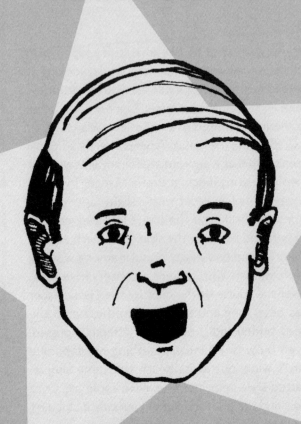

COOL
RATING

COMBOVER

For those that don't know when to call it a day and shave their head, the Combover stands as a shameful tribute to misplaced optimism and kidding yourself you've still got your mojo. In the classic Combover, the hair is worn short on the back and sides, bar a handful of thin strands that are grown long enough to be combed from one side of the head to another to cover up a bald pate. More of a situation you find yourself in than a deliberate choice, you are deluded if you think that your Combover is fooling anyone. Despite this fact, the style remains a favourite with country vicars, physics teachers that should be on the sex offenders' register and overweight singletons in middle management. The Combover is definitely one left to the professionals and certainly best concealed under a hat on a blustery day, lest your guilty – and painfully obvious secret – be revealed by a sudden gust of wind.

✂ Try to look like you don't have a Combover
✂ Try not to look like you've got a Combover

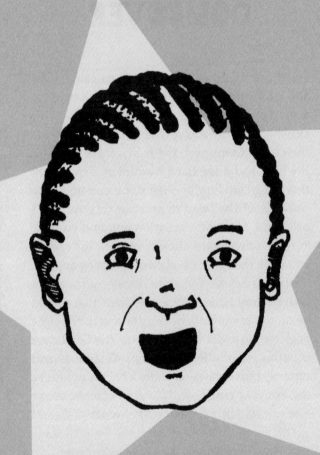

COOL
RATING

CORNROWS

If you own a large American car with a hydraulic system that allows it to bounce up and down, then you may also be considering Cornrows. Cornrows originated in sub-Saharan Africa but have since been popularised by African and Hispanic communities in the US. The style sees the hair braided into a series of tight French-braid-like rows that cling to the head and travel down the neck, sometimes finishing in thin beaded plaits. Cornrows can be created in straight lines or in complex geometric shapes, and when in place they are remarkably low maintenance. Since the 1970s this groovy style has been popular with rappers, models and those seeking to make their African roots apparent to anyone who hasn't noticed their garish tie-dye shirt, gourd and leather African pride necklace. A word of warning for anyone who does not have naturally curly hair: Cornrows are unbelievably time consuming and uncomfortable to knot in. But that pain is nothing compared to the agony and potential hair loss of trying to comb them out, and no amount of weed is going to make a weeping, partially bald white man look cool.

✂ Try to look like **Snoop Dogg**
✂ Try not to look like **Sean Paul**

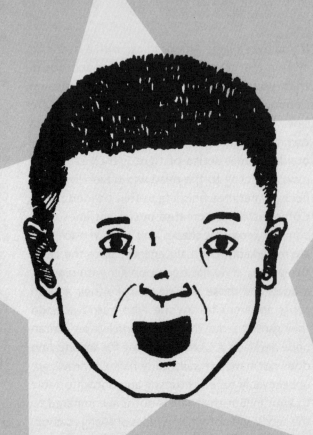

COOL
RATING

CREW CUT

If you are the kind of man who wants to look like he can yomp 20 miles when he actually gets breathless walking up a flight of stairs, then the Crew Cut is for you. Popularised by elite military units across the world, the Crew Cut, also known as the Jar Head or the High and Tight, is a no-nonsense 'do that screams attitude. From the jungles of Da Nang to the beaches of Normandy, this brutally short on top and shaved on the back and sides hairstyle is the trim of choice for both highly trained soldiers preparing to go into combat and physically imperfect, video game-playing loners who wish they were going with them. While eminently practical – not least as you could effectively create one with a penknife – what sporting a Crew Cut really says about you is that you're ready for action; whether it's storming a Taliban stronghold outside Kandahar, or paint-balling with the rest of the IT team in Aylesbury.

- ✄ Try to look like **Matt Damon** in *The Bourne Identity*
- ✄ Try not to look like **John Goodman** on *The Big Lebowski*

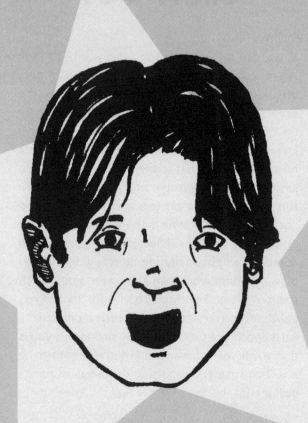

COOL
RATING

CURTAIN CUT

The Curtain Cut was made famous in the 1990s when the sloppy informality of this schoolboy 'do was popularised by a young, lisping David Beckham. It quickly became the crop of choice for men who had straight to wavy hair but who were beset by the kind of crippling shyness that made them want to hide behind their bangs when they talked to girls. The Curtain Cut is created by keeping the hair reasonably short and neat at the back and sides but allowing a long fringe to grow on the top, which is then divided, with either a middle or a side parting, and left to hang heavily on either side of the face (like a pair of curtains). The boyish look it inspires is strictly one for the youngsters, not least as an older man's hair is likely to be dryer and less flexible, so you'll end up looking like a scarecrow. On the plus side, this cut is perennially attractive to teenage girls; unfortunately this trait is usually wasted, as its classroom-based wearers are too afraid to talk to them anyway.

✂ Try to look like **Johnny Depp**
✂ Try not to look like **Worzel Gummidge**

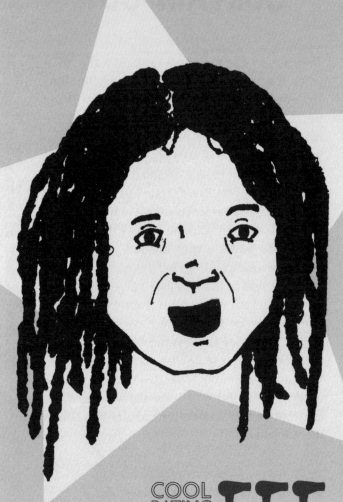

COOL
RATING 🔨🔨🔨

DREADLOCKS

Jah rastafari! Dreadlocks are a long, flowing mane of tightly wound bangs, popular with Rastafarians, trustafarians and street drinkers who haven't seen the inside of a shower for months. There are few hairstyles more synonymous with a type of music (reggae) and a laidback lifestyle than Dreadlocks. By letting your dreads grow out you tell the world you're a peace-loving vegetarian who is deeply committed to the consumption of marijuana in industrial quantities. The style is created when the hair is 'dreadlocked' into individual sections, either by back-combing, braiding, hand-rolling, or even allowing the hair to naturally 'lock' on its own. While Dreadlocks can vary in size, tidiness, and length, they should always look like they have been knitted by the wearer's grandmother, rather than fashioned deliberately in a salon. Despite being relatively easy to grow, dreads are one for the professionals. If you are a practising member of the Rastafarian faith, then they are a no brainer, but if you went to Eton and your dad is the CEO of a FTSE 100 company, then – for all our sakes – approach with care.

✂ Try to look like **Bob Marley**
✂ Try not to look like **Newton Faulkner**

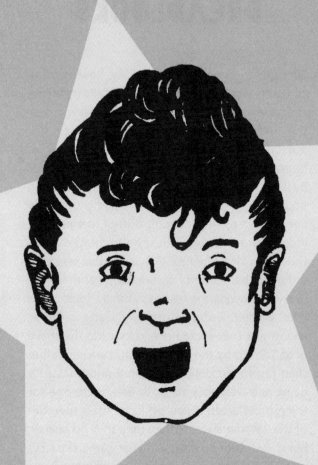

COOL
RATING

DUCKTAIL

Channelling the spirit of Eddie Cochran, Elvis and English teddy boys, the Ducktail was the first true rock 'n' roll hairstyle. Less charitably known as the DA (or Duck's Arse), the style is essentially based around long hair which is loaded with grease and then combed back around the sides of the head until it shines like wet liquorish. The comb is then used to define a central parting running from the crown to the nape at the back of the head, where the hair curls up, resembling the rear end of a duck. The fringe at the front of the head can be left either deliberately messy, so that untidy strands hang down over the forehead, or combed into a single 'elephant's trunk' which hangs down rebelliously across the forehead. Sporting a Ducktail harks back to a bygone era of drive-ins, soda fountains, crepe-soled shoes and bad teeth. If you are a proponent of the DA, you are either a free-wheeling roustabout who likes to settle their grievances with a switch-blade and a bicycle chain, or a grossly overweight driving instructor who spends their weekends at rockabilly revival events at Butlins in Skegness.

✂ Try to look like **Elvis**
✂ Try not to look like **Ted Bovis** from *Hi Di Hi*

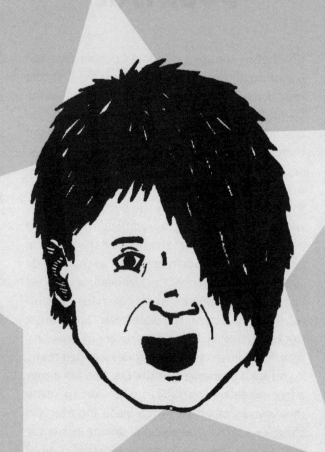

COOL
RATING

EMO

If you are a semi-suicidal loner in full-time education with quite pale skin, some tattoos inspired by the Mexican Day of the Dead and deep feelings of alienation from mainstream society, then you're likely to be seriously considering an Emo Cut. The Emo Cut tends to be dyed black, straightened and usually worn very long with an obligatory fringe falling over the eyes. This basic template is sometimes accessorised with some spiky bits, random splurges of bright colour, highlights or asymmetrical lines; in short, it's a hideous mish-mash of styles thrown together to indicate a kind of tortured creativity. Basically if you're rocking an Emo Cut you're trying to make sure your 'do looks like it absolutely wasn't done by your mum. More of a way of life than a haircut, the Emo Cut lets you show your inner pain on the outside – in hair form. Even better, it will mean that your parents will be embarrassed to walk down the same side of the street as you. The Emo Cut, like most teenage fads, is a passing treat, so enjoy it while you can. Besides, with all that home-grown dyeing, crimping and back-combing you'll be bald by the time you're 40.

✂ Try to look like **Pete Wentz** of Fall Out Boy
✂ Try not to look like **Edward Scissorhands**

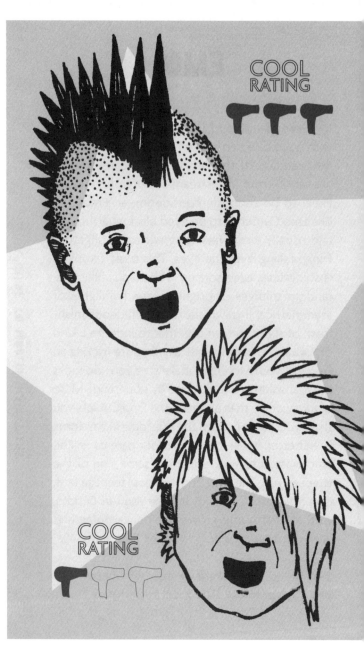

MOHAWK/ FAUXHAWK

The Mohawk is often associated with punk rockers but has a rich history reaching back to the Iroquis Indians in North America. The name is given to any hairstyle that is shaved on the sides to leave a strip of hair running down the middle of the head. This can be left natural, like a lifeless caterpillar, or combed upwards and spiked with to create a fin of varying lengths. It has many modern variants: Dreadhawks, Frohawks and Deathhawks are all flavours of the same pensioner-rattling style.

A Fauxhawk is where a single fin of hair is created across the top of the head by combing the hair upwards and together before fixing it with product, thus creating an imitation of a Mohawk. The name for this half-arsed attempt is created by combining the French word '*faux*' meaning false, with the English word 'Mohawk' meaning 'psycho's hair-cut'. One of the basic rules of good hairstyling is to find a look that suits you, and do it properly, so wearing the 'Fauxhawk' will never satisfy.

✂ Try to look like **Mr T**
✂ Try not to look like **Jack Osbourne**

A GUIDE TO MODERN HAIRSTYLES

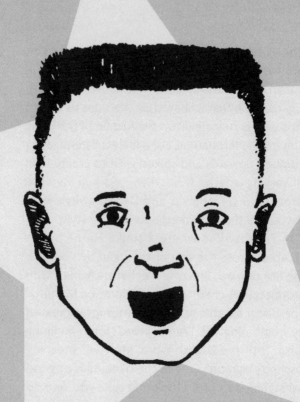

COOL
RATING

FLATTOP

If you're the kind of person who likes to combine a love of double-entry bookkeeping with the ability to balance a drink on top of your head, then the Flattop is for you. The Flattop is similar to the Crew Cut, bar the fact that the hair on the top of the head is deliberately styled to stand up about an inch, and levelled off to be flat. The 'do requires work with electric clippers to cut the hair close to the scalp, while the top is finished with scissors, sometimes utilising a special levelling comb to help create a horizontal plane. The hair is then blow-dried or waxed to stand up straight. It's worth noting that the egg-like shape of a human head means a spot on the crown will come close to being shaved to achieve the effect – this is known as the 'landing strip'. Beware, the Flattop is a high-maintenance option that needs weekly care to keep it in shape. The end result looks and feels like a trip to the headmaster's office which has made it enduringly popular with military veterans, policemen and anyone who routinely wears a short-sleeve shirt and tie to work.

✂ Try to look like **Dolph Lundgren** in *Rocky IV*
✂ Try not to look like **Simon Cowell**

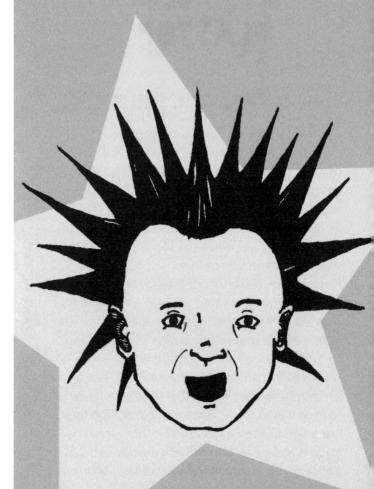

COOL
RATING

LIBERTY SPIKES

If you want a crazy 'do that makes you instantly recognisable, unable to wear a hat and deeply unpopular in crowded cinemas, then Liberty Spikes may be for you. The hair is grown out long and formed into large separate spikes using gel, soap or hairspray, or all three at the same time. Commonly associated with punk rock, Liberty Spikes actually date back to the Ancient Britons, whose warriors washed their long dark hair in lime water and packed it with clay to create the style. Back then it was worn as a badge of honour after they had killed an enemy; nowadays you won't have to kill anyone to get Liberty Spikes – though you may end up looking like you're seriously considering it.

✂ Try to look like **Benji Madden**
✂ Try not to look like **Sonic the Hedgehog**

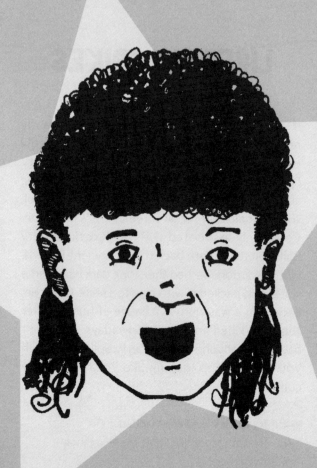

COOL
RATING ▼▼▼

MULLET

The Mullet is probably the most iconic haircut of the last twenty years. It is the term used to describe almost any hairstyle that is short at the front and long at the back. You don't need to be a former Radio One DJ, a trucker in the American Midwest or a football-loving casual with a whispy moustache to appreciate this righteous rug: the Mullet has it all. Balancing the masculine elements of the Crew Cut with the feminine charms of long, shoulder-length hair, it is both neat and casual at the same time and can be truly described as 'business in the front, party in the back'. Although there are references to Mullet-style cuts as far back as Roman times, it was not until the 1990s that the trim got a name, thanks to the American rap rock band the Beastie Boys. Perhaps the reason this iconic 'do went unchristened for so long is that this bi-level cut has very few other defining requirements and hereby lies its enduring strength. (Also called Ape Drape, Bi-Level, Beaver Paddle, Soccer Rocker, Squirrel Pelt, Hockey Hair and Tennessee Top Hat.)

✂ Try to look like **Chuck Norris**
✂ Try not to look like **Dog the Bounty Hunter**

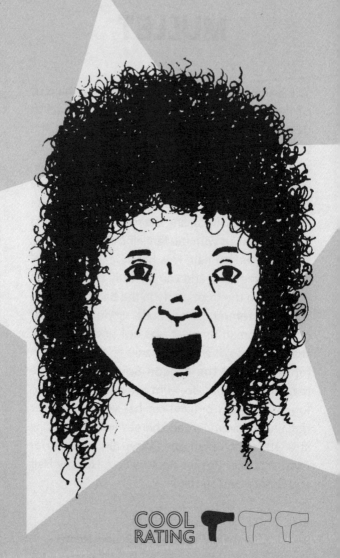

COOL
RATING

POODLE CUT

For people with straight or wavy hair, tight natural curls are something to envy. But the secret known only to those who are born with it is that curly hair is a curse that is about as style-able as a privet hedge and it will be treated by hairdressers accordingly. The result is that those 'blessed' with curly locks face a lifetime of alternating between boring Crew Cuts or looking like their head has boiled over. The paucity of options for the pube head only serves to make the popularity of the permanent wave among men in the mid-1980s all the more inexplicable. Throughout history, men and women have curled their hair with hot irons, but it was the creation of the acid perms in the 1970s that kicked off a craze for long curly hair that made a generation of rock stars and professional sportsman a laughing stock.

✂ Try to look like **Magnum PI**
✂ Try not to look like a member of **Def Leppard**

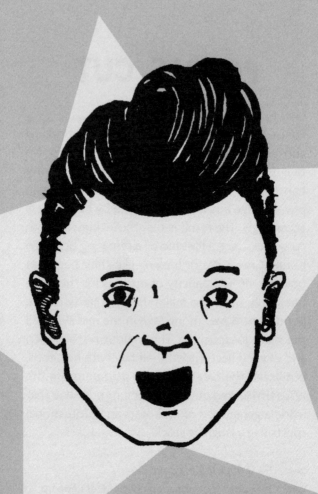

COOL
RATING ▼▼▼

QUIFF

If you fancy yourself as a dandy without the dandruff, then nothing is more untouchable than the timeless elegance of the Quiff. Favoured by Hollywood legends, male models and fresh-faced public school boys, the Quiff combines the pompadour hairstyles of the 1950s with elements of the Flattop and the skyward leanings of a Mohawk. Essentially you're looking at a fairly conservative trim at the back and sides, that loses all sense of decorum on top as the hair is grown long at the front, combed straight, then drawn high over the head and blown dry to create a mighty wave that looks like you've got a seagull sitting on your bonce. A tribute to lustrous hair growth, enduring style and the architectural powers of hair products, the Quiff is best shown off while singing Sinatra in a smoky jazz club or leaning on a stationary Harley Davidson while parked outside the local girls' secondary school.

✂ Try to look like **Alex Turner** from the Arctic Monkeys

✂ Try not to look like **Nick Grimshaw**

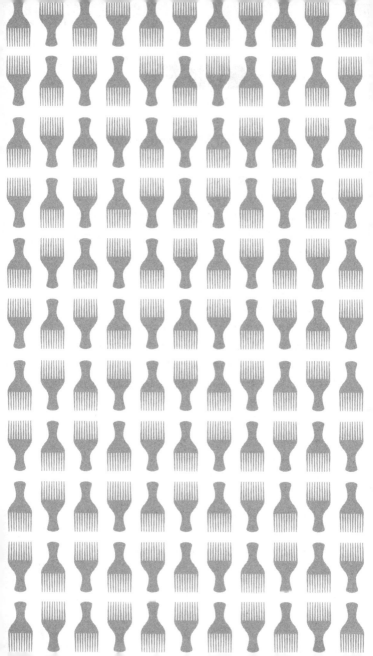

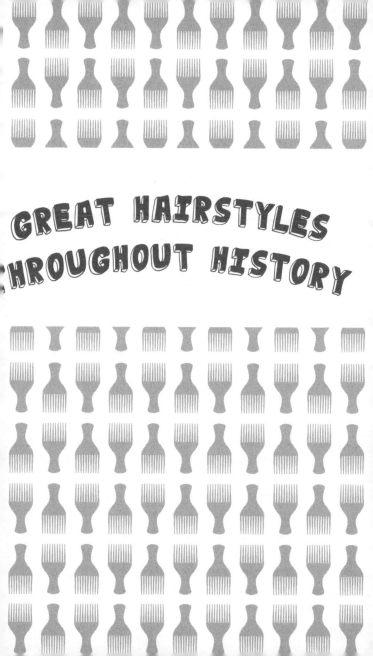

GREAT HAIRSTYLES
THROUGHOUT HISTORY

The relationship between a man and his mane has always been defined by the styling of his head garden. From the flowing curls of Sir Issac Newton to the untamed frizz of Albert Einstein, great men have always defined themselves as much by what's on their head, as what's in it. Here we look at some great men throughout history and how their 'do defined their destiny.

Albert Einstein

Albert Einstein was a German-born theoretical physicist who is best known as the creator of the world's most famous equation: $E = mc^2$. His life was defined by two immense breakthroughs. The first was a general theory of relativity which effected a revolution in modern physics, and the second was a crazy, flyaway hairstyle that became the benchmark for the 'mad scientist' look.

Einstein grew up largely in Switzerland. In school he achieved average grades in most subjects but excelled at mathematics and physics before going on to enrol in a four-year mathematics and physics teaching diploma in Zurich aged just 17. Bar a short spell in the Swiss Patent Office,

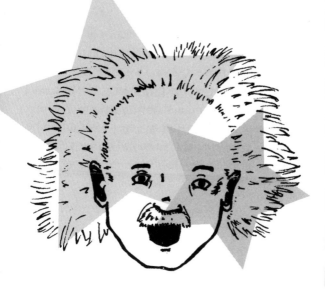

Einstein continued to break academic boundaries, completing his PhD and publishing four ground-breaking papers in 1905 alone. In 1921 he received the Nobel Prize in Physics for his services to theoretical physics, work that was pivotal in establishing both quantum theory and Einstein as the leading thinker of his generation. It was at this point that Einstein began to travel the world and – literally – let his hair down.

Following his immigration to the US in 1933, Einstein's trademark shock of grey hair became almost as famous as his work. Despite publishing more than 300 scientific papers along with over 150 non-scientific works, the great man is still best remembered for his hairstyle, which in all its flyaway, wiry and wild glory, was widely used in depictions of scientific genius in books, TV and film.

At the height of his popularity Einstein was often stopped on the street by people wanting an explanation of his theory. Legend has it that he would unconvincingly try to tell his fans, 'Sorry! Always I am mistaken for Professor Einstein.' Like anyone else ever looked like that ...

Andy Warhol

Andy Warhol was an American artist and a leading figure in pop art, a movement that challenged the traditions of fine art by including imagery from popular culture such as advertising, film and television. After starting life as a commercial illustrator, Warhol became a renowned and sometimes controversial artist, working in paint, print, photography, sculpture, film and even music. His studio, The Factory, was a famous gathering

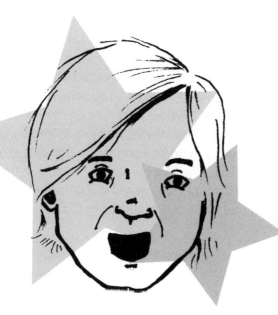

place in New York that brought together not just artists, but intellectuals, drag queens, playwrights, drug addicts and celebrities. His creations are enduring, popular and highly sought after and have become extremely valuable. The highest price ever paid for a Warhol is US$100 million for the painting 'Eight Elvises'.

It is a well-known fact that Warhol's famous silver Emo shock cut was actually a wig. Warhol had begun to wear wigs in the '50s, when he prematurely lost his hair and went grey. These grey and silver creations sat uneasily upon the artist's head, making him instantly recognisable. The hairpieces quickly became less of a fashion statement and more of an extension of the Warhol brand.

By the end of his life Warhol owned hundreds of wigs. He never threw one away and when he died in 1987, they were found in an assortment of boxes in his house. There are forty such specimens alone held in the Andy Warhol Museum in Pittsburgh. While it is easy to interpret such a hoarding as an act of madness, Warhol always had an eye for a potential money spinner and in 2006, a Warhol wig was sold for $10,800 at auction by Christie's.

Oscar Wilde

Oscar Wilde was an Irish writer and poet whose talent and dandyism made him one of the best-known personalities of his day. The son of Irish intellectuals, Wilde read classics at Oxford, where he became involved in the new philosophy of aestheticism, before relocating to London in 1878. A larger-than-life character, he moved in fashionable London circles where he published poems, lectured in the US and worked as a

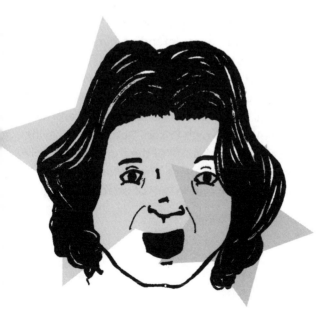

journalist. He became renowned for his sarcastic, cutting wit, flamboyant dress sense and long, thick hair, which he wore in a heavy set of centrally parted Curtains. When asked to explain reports that he had been seen on Piccadilly carrying a lily with his long hair flowing behind him, he replied, 'It's not whether I did it or not that's important, but whether people believed I did it.'

He became one of the country's most popular playwrights in the early 1890s, with a string of hits on the London stage like *Lady Windermere's Fan*, *A Woman of No Importance* and *The Importance of Being Earnest*. But the good times couldn't last and a run-in with amateur pugilist and professional Scottish misery-guts, the Marquis of Queensberry, saw Wilde in court defending himself against accusations of sodomy (which was then illegal). Wilde lost the subsequent Crown prosecution and had his health, hairdo and finances shattered by a spell enduring 'hard labour, hard fare and hard bed' in Wandsworth Prison. Despite still having time to bang out his side of the story in the deeply depressing masterpiece *The Ballard of Reading Gaol*, he died in exile in Paris of cerebral meningitis.

Paul McCartney

Sir Paul McCartney is a singer, songwriter and composer who achieved worldwide fame as a member of the Beatles and later with his own more rubbish band, Wings. *The Guinness Book of World Records* credits McCartney as the 'most successful composer and recording artist of all time', with sixty gold discs, and sales of over 100 million albums, but says nothing of his role in the creation of one of the most iconic haircuts of the 1960s.

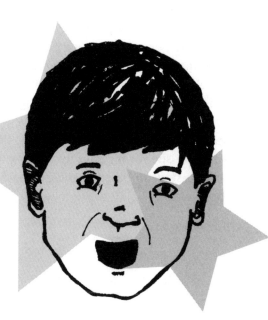

The Beatle haircut, also known as the Moptop (because of its resemblance to a mop), is a straight-cut, collar-length style with a long fringe. Legend has it that it is based on a look inadvertently created by Jürgen Vollmer who bumped into Lennon and McCartney after he had gone swimming and forgotten to style his hair. In his typically low-key way, McCartney described this pivotal moment in a 1979 radio interview: 'We saw a guy in Hamburg whose hair we liked. We asked him to cut our hair like he cut his.' The rest is history.

McCartney and his Moptop went on to become a worldwide sensation. The cut was widely imitated by screaming teens between 1964 and 1966. At the height of Beatlemania toy manufacturers began to produce plastic 'Beatle Wigs' in homage to the style, and even launched a 'Flip your Wig' board game based around it.

For his part, McCartney has kept roughly the same simple cut for most of his career, bar a few variations in length to suit the fashion of the times. Nowadays he spends his days lip syncing 'Hey Jude' at vast, stadium-based opening ceremonies around the world.

Hunter S. Thompson

Born in Louisville, Kentucky, to a middle-class family, Thompson went off the rails early and never formally graduated from school. Instead the American journalist and author served in the United States Air Force, where he developed a lifelong love of strong booze and even stronger writing. He became internationally famous with the publication of *Hell's Angels: The Strange and Terrible Saga of the Outlaw Motorcycle Gangs*

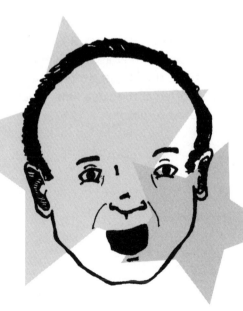

but became a legend when he created 'Gonzo' journalism with the publication of the seminal drug epic *Fear and Loathing in Las Vegas: A Savage Journey to the Heart of the American Dream* in 1972. Despite his chops as a political journalist and writer, he is perhaps better known for his love of whisky, drugs, cars, weapons and weird mayhem, and he duly devoted most of the second half of his life to indulging in them. Unusually for a counter-culture icon synonymous with freewheeling hippie youth, Thompson was no oil painting, but a perennial homebody and as bald as a coot. Yet his trademark Combover became as much a part of the 'Gonzo' look as his cigarette holder, sunglasses and Gladstone bag full of dangerous narcotics. A conventional/ unconventional look that allowed him to cavort with politicians, the literati, strippers and even policemen – often at the same time – seemingly without arousing suspicion.

'Rowdy' Roddy Piper

Roderick 'Roddy' George Toombs is better known by his ring name, 'Rowdy' Roddy Piper. The wrestler, chat-show host and film actor is known as one of the greatest heels (villains) in professional wrestling and was a leading star in the WWF between 1984 and 1996. Although he is actually Canadian, Rowdy was billed as coming from Scotland and was known for the kilt he wore in the ring, bagpipe entrance music and – at the

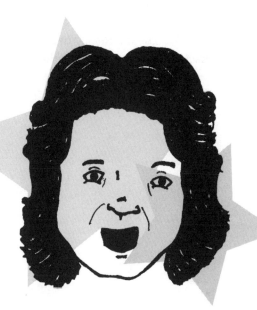

height of his fame – a luxurious Mullet that struck the fear of God into his opponents. He earned the nickname 'Rowdy' by displaying his trademark 'Scottish' rage and quick wit on camera. Such wit was on display during an episode of *Piper's Pit*, his long-running WWF chat show, when Piper interviewed Fijian wrestler Jimmy Snuka. Rowdy tried to make Snuka 'feel at home', by offering him bananas and coconuts, a gesture that was immediately misinterpreted by the bulky islander. In the ensuing melee, Piper smashed a coconut shell over Snuka's head causing the Fijian to rampage through the studio, destroying much of the set. Rowdy then threw his guest to the ground and – Ape Drape flowing in the wind – shoved a banana down his guest's throat before leaving through a back door. Move over Jonathan Ross.

Adolf Hitler

Adolf Hitler was the architect of the Holocaust, the instigator of the Second World War and an all-round bad egg. His theories of racial purity and a return to medieval Teutonic values were instrumental in the dramatic rise and fall of the Third Reich and in the creation of what historians now agree is the world's most uptight haircut.

Despite ruling Germany, Hitler was actually born in Austria. His experiences serving in

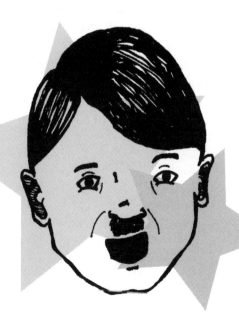

the trenches during the First World War and Germany's subsequent capitulation, combined with his incarceration for his political views and years trying to make it as a painter, all fuelled an inner rage against the established German nobility that drove him to create the Nazi state. He was Chancellor of Germany from 1933 to 1945 and dictator of Nazi Germany (as Führer und Reichskanzler) from 1934 to 1945, during which time he sported a haircut so severe it made grown men wince just to look at it. Shorn close at the back and sides with a thin greased smear of dark black hair pulled to the side of a razor-sharp parting, Hitler's 'do became as evocative of the era as mass rallies, over-dramatic speeches and casual anti-Semitism.

Things may have turned out differently had Hitler worn a head of long golden curls but we will never know as the world's most evil man took his own life just before the fall of Berlin in 1945.

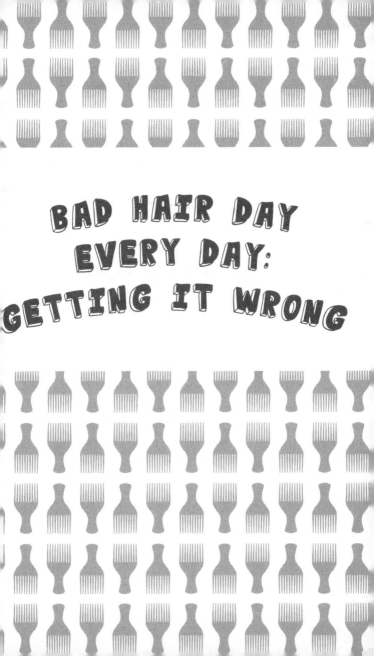

BAD HAIR DAY EVERY DAY: GETTING IT WRONG

Have you woken up with a head like a toilet brush? Maybe you have just attended a job interview looking like an onion, or have gone on a date with hair that looks and smells like a dead sheep. If so you're having a bad hair day (BHD). Here are some tips that should stop your BHD becoming a bad hair week.

Avoiding Bad Hair Days

For most men bad hair days are like bad relationships: everybody has at least one but if you're lucky they won't last long. As your best bet is to try to get your rug looking righteous before you leave the house, here is our five-point guide to making the most of what you've got.

Wash and Style your Hair Regularly

Any day you leave the house with dirty or oily hair is not going to turn out well. Clean, healthy hair is the basis of all good-looking hairstyles, so wash your hair regularly. This means at least twice a week.

Restyling your 'do from scratch each morning is probably the most effective way to achieve a great hairstyle every time. It is best if you start working on your rug when it is wet; if you don't have time to shower in the morning, wash it the night before and then wet it again with water the next day.

One word of warning – don't go to bed with wet hair or you'll end up looking like you've been sleeping in a wind tunnel.

Don't Scrimp on Products

When it comes to styling your hair, avoid cheap gel or mousse. They will flake leaving dandruff, make your hair greasy and their hold is less likely to last. Spending a couple of quid more on quality products is also economical as you won't need to use as much. Finally, only re-apply your product when you have to; you may find that a little water and some coaxing will work just as well.

Mix & Match Shampoos & Conditioners

It seems odd but your hair can gradually become accustomed to your shampoo and conditioner over time, so they will become less effective. Switch your shampoo and conditioner routine every few months to give it a boost. You may even find that you draw inspiration from a new scent and texture.

Change your Style

If your head gear looks bad more days than it looks good, it is probably time for a serious rug rethink. This could simply be changing the side you part or it could be investing in a full makeover from your stylist.

Keep it Short

It may seem like cheating, but keeping your hair short is the easiest way to keep BHDs to a minimum. Short hair also means more haircuts, a more defined style and fewer split ends. Easy!

Top Ten Worst Celebrity Hairstyles

We are a nation obsessed with celebrities. Whether they're rolling out of Soho House at 3 a.m., hiding behind giant sunglasses in the duty free shop at Heathrow Airport, or kicking a hapless photographer in the kneecaps, we lap up their every move.

Like it or not, we spend so much time reading about every detail of the lives of celebrities that it is inevitable we will start to copy them. For some this might mean taking a Caribbean holiday, buying a designer handbag or sliding behind the wheel of a quarter-million-pound Bentley, but for most of us ordinary Joes the entry-level mode of celebrity emulation will be a new haircut.

But get real ... because a haircut custom designed for a heavily made-up celebrity with the body of a Greek god is going to look like a car crash on your pasty, overweight form down the pub. Even worse, celebrities are guilty of some of the worst crimes against hairdressing ever perpetrated and to emulate them would be sartorial suicide. While we realise that for some true fans these words will fall on deaf ears, in the interest of saving the rest of you, here is our list of the top ten worst celebrity haircuts. Handle with care.

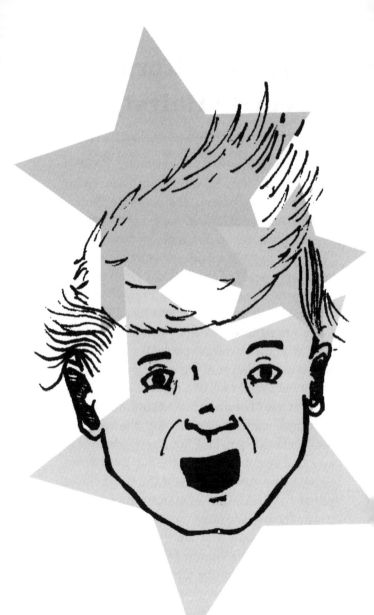

Donald Trump's Flyaway Rug

The unique hair do of the business mogul and *Apprentice* host, Donald Trump, defies not only good taste but also gravity. Dubbed affectionately as the Cotton Candy Combover, it combines a poor attempt to cover baldness with a swoop of hair that looks remarkably like a toupee and a dash of steadfast refusal to let go of the few remaining wisps of hair left on his head (which flutter in the wind like broken antennae). Not that the sheer ridiculousness of Trump's haircut has slowed him down. On the contrary, Trump is worth some $2.9 billion and is now married for the third time, to a former swimwear model twenty years his junior, a woman who can no doubt see through the 'do to the billionaire property developer's more tangible assets.

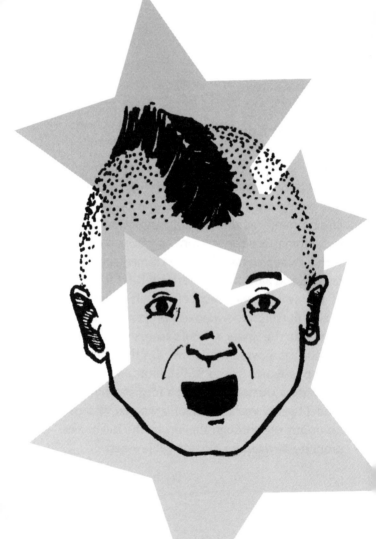

David Beckham's Floppy Mohawk

For those who follow such things, the dress sense of part-time footballer and full-time clothes horse David Beckham must present something of an enigma. On one hand a dedicated follower of fashion, on the other, never more than a red carpet away from turning up looking like a tattooed circus clown. In Beckham's defence he never stays with one style for long so faux pas are quickly forgotten. He remains equally schizophrenic when it comes to his barnet. He has sported Buzz Cuts, '20s-style flops, Mullets, spikes and greased DAs, sometimes all in the same magazine. However, the floppy Mullet he wore on the first day of his arrival at LA Galaxy looked more like he was recovering from recent brain surgery than setting trends. Perhaps, like his football, David has realised he is now famous enough to get by without really trying.

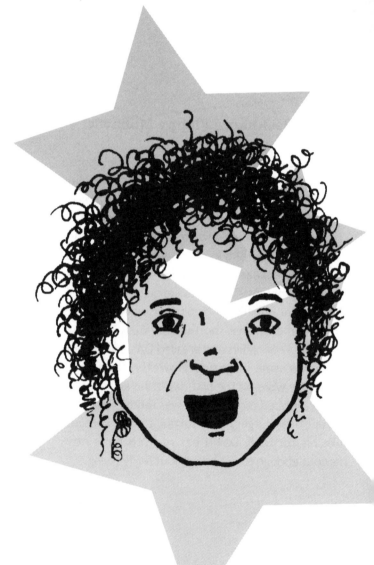

Mick Hucknall's Curly Fringe

Arguably the Simply Red lead singer was dealt a terrible double blow when the follicle gods issued him with both flaming red hair and a tight head of curls. Despite being the son of a barber, Hucknall did nothing to address this situation when he first came to fame in the 1980s. Instead he chose to sport a single vomit of long curly fringe which cascaded from beneath an affected flat cap like a spaniel's ear. By the 1990s the podgy-faced crooner had swapped the fringe for sex addiction and equally objectionable Dreadlocks before settling down to his current sedate waves.

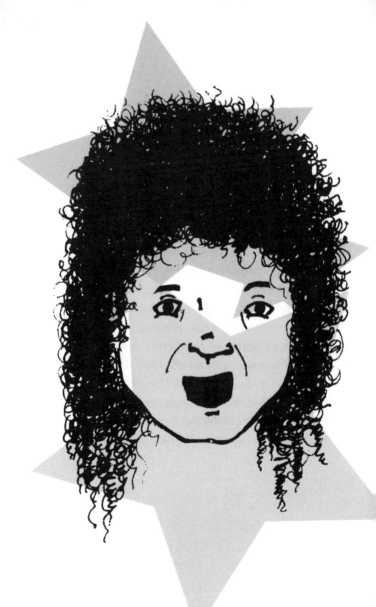

Brian May's Poodle Cut

With a role playing lead guitar for one of the world's greatest rock groups, a CBE for charity work and a PhD in astrophysics, Brian May has got a lot going for him. Unfortunately all of these achievements are totally overshadowed by his infamous Poodle haircut. While this tress travesty may have made sense in the drug-enhanced '70s, to the modern eye his generous curls, worn untamed and beyond the shoulder, seem more like the self-effacing axe man is being attacked by a swarm of bees than expressing himself artistically.

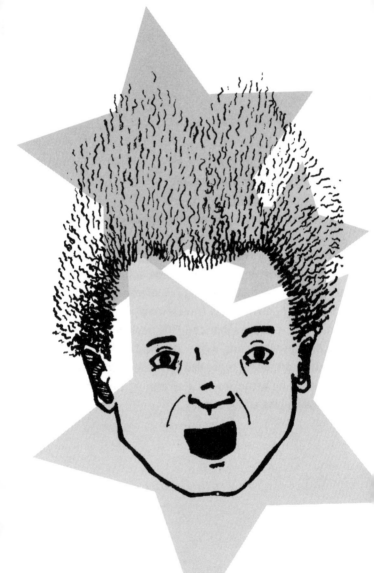

Don King's Frizz Tower

Don King's crazy Frizz job has become as much of a permanent fixture at the ring-side celebrations in Vegas as raised fists, swollen eyes and tearful dedications to the protective powers of Jesus Christ. The back-combed tower of Afro fuzz sitting on top of King's smiling face seems to have developed some time between his release from prison (for murder) in 1970 and his journey to Zaire to promote the Ali-Foreman, Rumble in the Jungle fight of 1974, and has kept on growing ever since. Now frosted with grey, it's still a style that makes it clear simultaneously that King is, a) as mad as a hatter and b) rich enough to just not care.

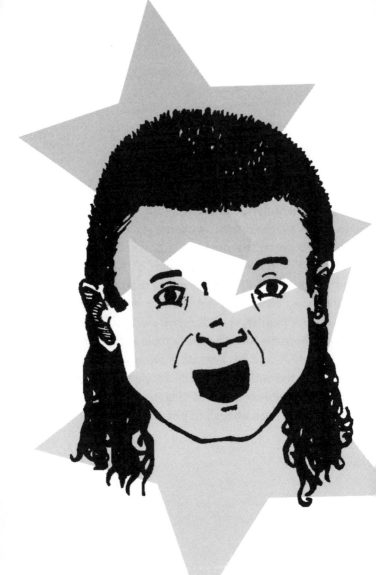

Billy Ray Cyrus' Mullet

It seems unlikely that Billy Ray Cyrus realised when he told his hairstylist to crop it short on top but leave the back, that his infamous Mullet would come to define all that's wrong with hairstyles, America, country music and the 1990s. Despite being widely ridiculed at the time, Cyrus's Mullet gave birth to a generation of misguided imitators. Cyrus at least wised up but it would take the Kentucky-born singer and actor a decade to outrun his bi-level barnet, eventually being reduced to turning his back on his honkytonk roots and becoming a Christian, before returning to the limelight on the Disney Channel as Hannah Montana's dad.

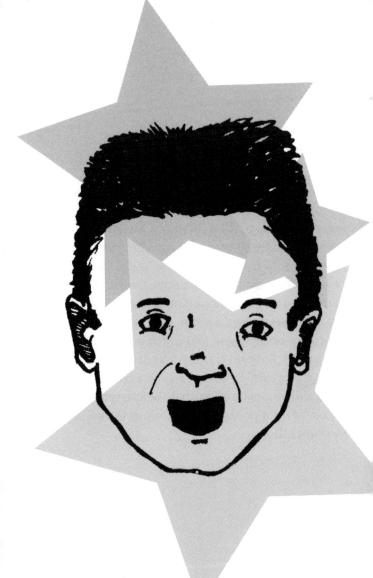

Simon Cowell's Flattop

Simon Cowell is the hugely successful A & R man, TV producer and entrepreneur behind some of the most toe-curlingly bad, yet inexplicably popular, music and television of the last ten years. Much of his fame as a television personality stems from his blunt criticism and borderline cruelty towards the deluded and talentless contestants on his various talent shows, as well as his astoundingly poor taste in music, clothing and haircuts. Cowell's trademark shapeless Box Cut serves the dual purpose of making Cowell look like an Easter Island statue and demonstrating exactly what happens when a man who has more money than Croesus chooses to spend no more than a tenner on a haircut.

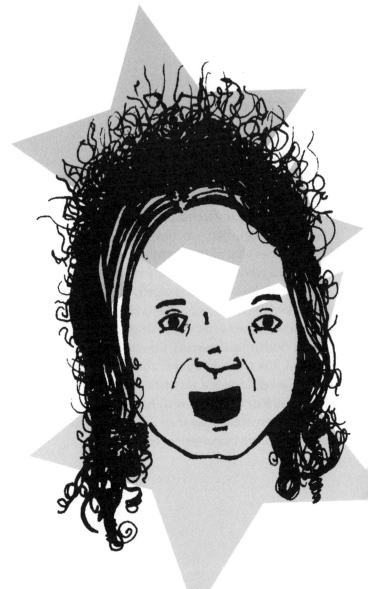

Russell Brand's Bird's Nest

Stand-up comedian and actor Russell Brand is as well known for his eccentric behaviour and outspoken views as he is for his ridiculous dress sense and baffling success with the ladies. If anyone over the age of 19 were to be seen in broad daylight wearing skin-tight jeans, pixie boots, three belts, two scarves and a dozen bangles, they would either have to have a million pounds in the bank or at the very least a decent haircut. Brand has the money but sadly his trademark back-combed bird's nest still stands out as one of the worst haircuts in Hollywood. In recent years, Brand has toned down the frizz, choosing instead a lank set of long Curtains, but rather than addressing the problem they make him look like a wet beagle.

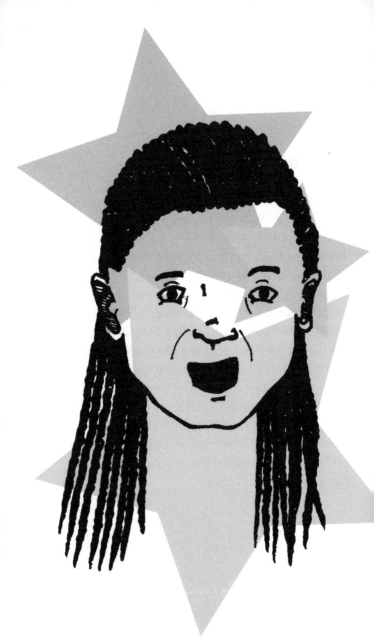

Axl Rose's Cornrows

Axl Rose is best known as the red-haired mentalist who came to fame as the lead singer of infamous LA hair metal band Guns n' Roses. At the apex of the band's success, Rose's fiery personality resulted in all of the band's original members leaving, possibly as a result of music differences but arguably due to the hideous woven Cornrow hairstyle the flame-haired singer had adopted. But you have to take your hat off to him: finding a hairstyle this offensive, in an era when highlights and back-combed manes for men were de rigueur, is quite an achievement. Rose spent the next ten years as a recluse, struggling to complete the next Guns n' Roses album *Chinese Democracy*, an effort which turned out – like his Cornrows – to be total crap.

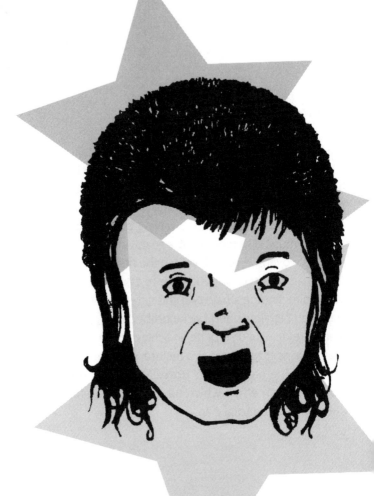

David Bowie's Fright Wig

David Bowie's track record for reinvention gives him probably the broadest coiffure canvas of any man on the planet. As the gender-bending rock star doesn't even have eyes the same colour, he soon realised that he could get away with wearing everything from a dress to a spacesuit without anyone calling him on it. To be fair, Bowie's various reincarnations usually hit the spot more than they miss, but his Ziggy era, red fright wig was truly a monstrosity, combining everything that's bad about dyeing your hair, styling your hair, and spiking your hair, to create a 'do that made him look like a frayed piece of rope. At the end of the day, it was only the welcome distraction provided by his off-the-shoulder, skin-tight jumpsuit that saved him from being lynched by the hairdressers of Great Britain.

Quick Fixes for Problem Hair

Nobody is perfect and most us are looking to do the best with the hand we've been dealt, whether it is a mane of tousled tresses as thick as velvet curtains, or a dusting of fine fuse-wire follicles that are rendered translucent by direct sunlight. Here are a few quick tips for making the most of your problem mop.

Fine or Thinning Hair

Thick, moisturising conditioners and heavy styling products are out. They will weigh down your hair strands and make them clump together to expose patches of skin on your scalp. Instead have your hair cut every three to four weeks. Try going for some shaggy layers that will help to create the illusion of greater thickness. As a last resort, a Crew Cut will most effectively blend areas of thinning hair in with the rest.

Oily or Greasy Hair

Overexposure to heat is always bad news. Too long under hot showers, the dreaded hair dryer, as well as vigorous brushing or combing, will all trigger unwelcome oil production on the scalp as the body tries to protect itself. Wash your hair in lukewarm water and try to use fewer strokes when brushing. This will reduce the amount of oil you distribute from your scalp to the hair. A good tip is to rinse your hair in lemon water after shampooing, as the acid helps to strip away excess oil build-up.

Dry or Brittle Hair

It's all about balance, so don't shampoo your 'do too frequently and avoid hot water. Wash your hair in lukewarm water no more than twice a week so you don't blast your hair's natural oils. In this case you are looking to make the most of your body's natural oils, so styling using a natural bristle brush will help to spread the goodness from your scalp down the length of the hair shaft.

Curly or Frizzy Hair

The ladies love curls but for the owner they can be a nightmare. Natural curls can easily become a horrible frizz if they dry out, so don't wash them too frequently, and don't indulge in vigorous towel drying. Instead wash twice a week in lukewarm water, use a good conditioner and blot your curls dry with a towel to add bounce to your bubbles rather than sending them into spasm.

Dandruff and Flaky Scalp

If you suffer from snow storms on the shoulders, daily shampooing and conditioning is important for removing flakes and keeping your scalp clean and moisturised. Be sure to rinse your hair thoroughly to clear any residue from it. Finally get out in the sun. Like all skin conditions, ultraviolet light can be effective in stimulating the skin to repair itself.

Dull or Lifeless Hair

Avoid any styling products which can be applied to wet hair, this means pomades and water-based unguents, as they will wash out your locks and leave them even limper. One tip is to massage beer into your hair a few times a week after shampooing, then rinse. The hops coat your hair and add volume and shine – plus you can drink what's left over.

All of the Above

There comes a time when every man has to admit defeat. Shave it all off or buy a decent hat.

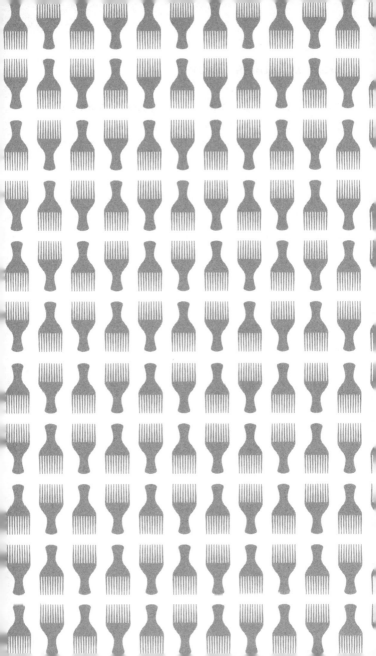

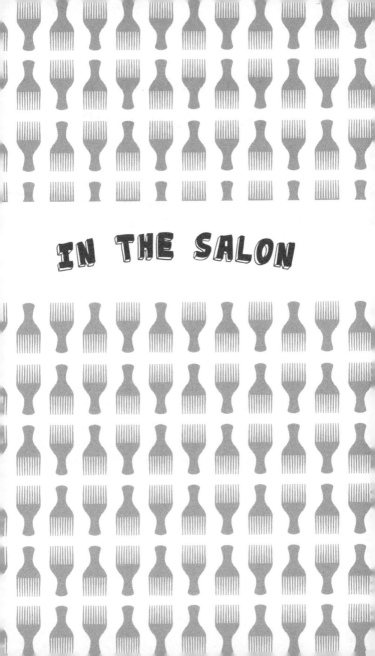

IN THE SALON

What Makes a Good Haircut?

It may come as a surprise, but the first step to getting great-looking hair is getting a grip on the basics of hairdressing. Knowing what goes into a haircut will help you think about how you can construct a look that kills. There are three key areas to focus on in the design of a good haircut:

1. The shaping
2. The blending
3. The finishing

You need to have a sense of what you want from each of these areas if you want to communicate with your barber or stylist and – more importantly – to know when to complain if your scissorsmith is not making the grade in front of the mirror.

The Shaping

You don't need to be Stephen Hawking to work out that the length and shape of your barnet can go a long way to defining the look of your entire head. A well-chosen haircut can help to draw the focus away from weak facial features and enhance your best ones. A bad 'do can make them look a whole lot worse. For example, a full, round Bowl Cut on a guy with a round face, will leave him looking more like a bowling ball than a member of The Stone Roses. While a lean-looking Flattop with defined square edges on the same round bonce, would add much-needed balance. If you want to make the most of what you've been given by Mother Nature, it is advisable that you think beyond fashion and choose the kind of haircut that compliments your face shape.

The Blending

A properly blended haircut will have no visible lines of where your hair changes in length. There should not be obvious tram lines in the hair created by your stylist, where he or she has been cutting it between their fingers. When viewed from the back, you should not see any dark (too thick) or light (too thin) spots (unless it's part of the style for some reason). From the front, there should be no random steps, sprouts on the crown or flyaway hairs. All this is doubly crucial with a short haircut. If your stylist has failed to blend properly, you will end up looking like you got drunk the night before and hacked at it yourself with a pair of kitchen scissors.

The Finishing

How a haircut is finished is critical to achieving a solid result. If you've ever wondered why old-school barbers spend twenty seconds shearing the top of your head and twenty minutes fiddling around your neck line with a razor, this is why. Years of experience has taught them that attention to detail while finishing can add polish to a so-so haircut, while sloppy finishing can make a good piece of work look like it was done by a 5-year-old. A properly finished haircut needs to meet the following criteria:

1. The outline of the haircut should follow the natural hairline as closely as possible or you'll end up looking like you're wearing an ill-fitting wig.
2. There should not be any hair sticking up at the crown or you'll end up looking like an onion.
3. Your haircut should look good with or without styling products.

For the record, styling products should be used to enhance a style, not create one. Unless you have a thing for looking like a Ken doll, you need to understand that a properly shaped, blended, and finished haircut should look killer with or without the goo.

How to get the Best out of your Stylist

If you've ever been on the business end of a bad haircut, you know that it can lead to weeks of ego-shattering embarrassment, that no amount of hair gel can conceal. A bad haircut almost always is blamed on the barber or stylist, but it's probably worth swallowing your pride and accepting that in some cases a proportion of that blame lies with you. Having unrealistic expectations, poor communication, or just being an unfriendly sod, can all lead to a rug crisis that will see you wearing a baseball cap for a month.

Here are a few tips on communicating with your barber or stylist that may help you leave the salon looking more like George Clooney than Robert Smith.

1. Be Selective

Find a cutter who specialises in the kind of style that suits you, and stick with them. How do you find such a person? Swallow your masculine pride and ask around. You would have no problem asking your friends where they got a kick-ass pair of trainers, or who sold them their car, so how about widening the search to their hair? Find someone who has a haircut similar to the one you're after and just ask them who did it. Easy!

2. Book your Appointment

As a general rule, salons and even traditional barbers which offer appointments will have a better customer service and be prepared to invest more time in getting what you want. By necessity, walk-in operations focus on volume of customers so they will need to do as many heads as they can, as quickly as they can – if you're looking for anything more than a short back and sides, this can lead to mistakes. An appointment ensures your stylist feels that they don't need to rush through your haircut, and allows you time to pay attention to the detail. Of course this is a two-way arrangement so you need to be on time for your appointment and shouldn't forget to call ahead if you're going to be late or cancel.

3. Don't be First and Don't be Last

Like anyone else, your friendly neighbour hair honcho will take a little time to get warmed up in the morning, so don't turn up when they're still trying to finish their decaf latte. Equally, arriving in the salon at one minute before closing and expecting a decent trim, when the stylist has just spent eight hours standing behind the chair, can result in some pretty poor cuts. As a rule, try to get a slot in the middle of the day. Not only will your stylist have had time to get their swerve on, many salons are slower in the middle of the day so they have more time to spend with you.

IN THE SALON

4. Be Nice

There's an unwritten rule that you should never anger hairdressers, tattoo artists and rabbis at a bris. Before they go to work on you, remember it costs you nothing to make an effort to be friendly to your stylist, and in turn it can pay dividends in the service you get. Being rude to the person cutting your hair may ruin their day, but a bad haircut will ruin your whole week.

5. Be Clean

This might sound like a no brainer but most stylists will prefer to work on hair that is clean and free of product. If you don't want to touch your hair, why would they? On a more practical point, showing up with clean hair that is free of products allows the stylist to see how it falls naturally and shape it accordingly.

6. Be Open to New Ideas

If they are any good, your stylist is trained to know how to make any old mop look good and any follicle jockey worth their salt should have a solid idea of which styles might best frame your face and enhance your features. When your cropper makes a suggestion, don't write it off, even if you have had the same cut for years. If you don't like the outcome, you can always grow it back.

7. Don't Expect Them to be Psychic

Psychologists tell us that when a message is communicated orally, only about 20 per cent of the instruction is understood accurately. Apply this to a haircut and you'll end up with some pretty interesting results, so why not make things simple and bring a photo of the style you want. The trend of bringing a photo to the salon has been around for a while but really came to prominence when tens of thousands of women began turning up at salons with pictures of Jennifer Aniston and demanding the – then unnamed – Rachel Cut. Men aren't great at expressing themselves as it is, so a photo could mean more than a thousand grunted words. Your stylist will appreciate the effort and will get a clear idea of what you want without having to read your mind.

8. Be Self Aware

If you're 18 stone with a head like a bucket of concrete, no hairstyle in the world is going to make you look like Robert Pattinson, so don't expect your cropper to work miracles. Using a male celebrity as a guide for the type of haircut you're after is fine, but it's important to be realistic. Chances are your stylist might be able to capture some of the nuances of your favoured style without replicating it. Invariably this is going to suit you better than a slavish copy.

9. Don't Forget to Tip

Whether you're getting a £10 trim in the train station, or £110 make-over in the West End, basic human psychology is at work here and barbers and stylists are almost always going to spend more time with clients who are good tippers than those who are not. Sorry skinflints.

A Guide to Men's Hair Products

For years there were only three choices when it came to men's styling products: a tub of Brylcreem, a dandruff-inducing green gel that looked and smelled like Swarfega, and 'men's hairspray', which was closer to a lacquer used to bond plywood than a hair product. Not surprisingly most of us gave them a wide berth.

Nowadays the market for men's styling products, shampoos and conditioners is booming, with hundreds of excellent products competing for shelf space. Gone are the days of just grabbing any old tub of gel and hoping for the best, because such are the styling options for men that even the trendy, 'just rolled out of bed' look takes a lot of work – and a good dollop of the right product.

You can divide styling products into two general categories: fixatives and pliables. Fixatives are things like gels and hairsprays that dry hard on the hair to hold it in shape. These are best used to style hair into unusual, spiky or geometric shapes. Pliables are things like waxes and pomades. These retain moisture to make the hair flexible and are best applied for more natural effects.

You should be looking to use a product that suits your hair type. This means that – unless you're creating an extreme style – you should look like you're not using any product at all. Choose something that adds shine without looking greasy, and shape without destroying the bounce and body of your barnet. You get the idea.

Fixatives

Gel

Gels are good for those who want shiny, sleek-looking hair. The cheap stuff you get in supermarkets tend to dry out and flake off, which makes you look like you've either got terminal dandruff or you've just been skiing (hard to argue in mid-summer), so it pays to get the good stuff. Gels usually come in a choice of firm or light hold. You may also get a choice of dry (normal) or wet look (shiny). As a guide, those with fine hair should use the lighter products, and those with thick hair will need the firmer hold to achieve the same effect.

The good news is that a quality gel is fairly robust and will 'remember' the shape you have crafted. So when your hair has dried, you can still comb through it to style and maintain the shape. Wet-look gel can also be 'reactivated' by wetting your hands and running them through the 'do to reset the style.

Hairspray

It's worth remembering that hairspray is a finishing, not styling, product. This means that it's designed to lock a style in place, rather than create it, so if you spray your hair before you start to style you are likely to end up with a tangled mess. As with gel, those with fine hair should choose lighter hold products for their locks, or they'll end up as matted strands. Having said that, the best results with hairspray are usually achieved by those with fine hair. It's worth noting that many hair sprays now contain a sunscreen which will protect any barnet from the dehydrating rays of the sun.

Pliables

Most pliables are wax, gum or water based and usually sold packed in a tub or tin. For best results with a pliable, you should apply a small amount to the palms of your hands and rub them together until your hands warm the product into a viscous liquid before applying it to slightly damp or dry hair.

Pomade

Pomade can be used to add shine while maintaining a flexible hold. It will give a wet, shiny look. While it can be used to give shine and separation to long hair, it is best suited for a sleek, well-groomed style reminiscent of the 1920s. Most pomades are pretty heavy, so they will make fine hair look greasy and limp. It is super important to wash this product out of your hair every night or it will accumulate on the scalp to create a flaky and possibly smelly result.

Wax

Waxes are similar to pomade, but are normally more aggressive and petroleum based. This product is great for lending shine and control to short cuts like Flattops and Buzz Cuts. Waxes are also good for managing very thick hair. Remember that oil and water don't mix so the product must be applied to a completely dry bonce. Again, remember to wash the product out at night, and never use a wax on fine hair unless you want to end up looking like your mates have deliberately glued your hair down.

Mud

A mud (or fibre) should only be used when maximum control is needed. It will give a more natural matte finish and is great for giving texture to short hair. If you want to create a deliberately messy bed-head style, reach for the mud.

Cream

A styling cream has the consistency of a soft, opaque wax. As these products are lighter, they are better for fine hair, can be particularly good at controlling flyaway hair, and can give a bit of shine and control to those who like to look like they haven't styled it at all (despite having spent forty-five minutes in front of the mirror before going out). If your hair is curly, a cream is a great option to add shine and keep your curls bouncy and defined.

How to Have Healthy Hair

Brace yourself because here comes some bad news: the hair on your head is dead. Yes, your mop is made up from nothing more than protein and keratin. It can't repair itself when it's damaged like other parts of your body. This means that once it is broken, the only option you have is to cut it off.

The good news is that you can keep your Fred Astaire maintained so it stays healthy looking for longer, but this means following some simple hair-care rules if you want to keep your tresses strong, flexible and shiny.

Use a Good Shampoo and Conditioner

Forget 2 in 1 blends – you need separate shampoo and conditioning routines. Inevitably, shampoo will take it out of your hair, so only apply the shampoo once in a session regardless of what it says on the bottle. A good shampoo will help clean the hair but can also help to reduce the loss of proteins and moisture. A good conditioner will further minimise this problem, as well as adding softness and shine. Gently combing conditioner through the hair will help to ensure equal coverage.

Cool it Off

Make no mistake, very hot water will strip many of the essential oils from the hair and dry out the scalp, so take it easy in the shower, lukewarm water only when shampooing and rinsing.

Pat it Dry

Towel drying is one of the biggest causes of damage to men's hair. There's no point treating your mop like a wet Labrador when you step out of the shower and still expect to look good. When hair is wet, it is highly susceptible to damage, and rubbing it vigorously can lead to frizziness and split ends. To properly towel your barnet dry, shake out the excess water and stroke your hair in the direction it grows with the clean, dry towel. It takes a bit longer this way but you really will notice the difference to its condition.

Don't Burn it

Blow drying is another incredibly common cause of irreversible damage to the hair. Excessive blow drying can dry out both the hair and scalp. The same goes for heating tongs, crimpers and irons. If you must use a blow dryer, you will need to protect your hair with a thermal styling spray and gently detangle it with a wide-toothed comb to ensure your tresses are dried evenly. Never blow the hair so it is bone dry – always leave it slightly damp if you want to avoid a mop like fried chicken.

Say No to Chemical Warfare

Over time colouring or perming your head garden will leave it damaged, dry, and dull. However, if you are going to do it then your best bet is to give home kits a miss and turn to your stylist for a touch up. Though professional treatments can be pricey, your stylist will know how to properly protect your hair and will choose the best products for your hair type. The bonus is that a stylist will almost always make the results look more natural so you won't end up looking like Roy Orbison.

Use the Right Tools for the Job

Though it's usually down to what comes out of the tap, soft water is easier on the hair. Don't use a brush on wet hair when the hair is most vulnerable, as it will create split ends. Finally when combing through wet hair, use a wide-toothed comb and gently work out any tangles. Always use clean, dry towels.

Healthy Body, Healthy Head

It may seem obvious but the condition of your hair is often a reflection of the overall health of your body. It may be annoying, but doing all those boring things that your personal trainer tells you (eat well, exercise, drink plenty of water, get enough sleep, and reduce stress in your life) will result in a healthier scalp and a better-looking barnet.

Ditch the Beanie

A tight hat (or even a ponytail) can cause a horrible-sounding condition known as 'traction alopecia', in which you pull your own hair out of your scalp. A tight tiffler can also cause breakage of the follicles and damage to the cuticles. Wear one for long enough and the damage can become permanent. Nasty.

Keep it Coiffed

Since the only real way to remove damaged hair is to cut off the damaged section, keeping your hair trimmed regularly will help eliminate split ends and the associated frizziness. Even if you're growing it out, make sure to get your Tony Blair trimmed about once every six weeks or so.

Soothe your Scalp

A good growth of hair starts from the scalp, so for a fringe that's strong, and shiny, make sure you take good care of your scalp with some light massage. This will increase blood flow to the skin and encourage growth. For the same reasons a little bit of scalp TLC is not a bad tip for those who are starting to go thin on top.

IN THE SALON

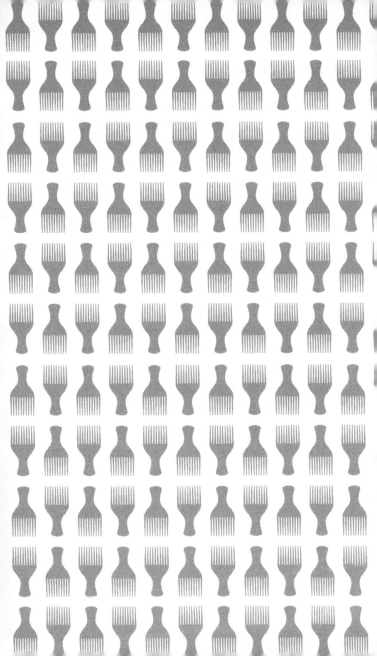

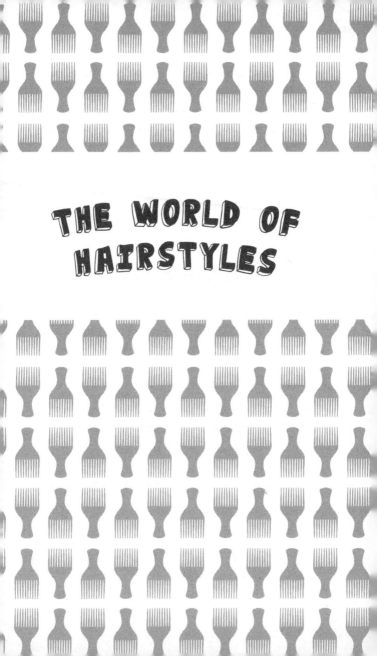

THE WORLD OF HAIRSTYLES

Okay, so you know that the hair on your head is dead material which consists mainly of a fibrous protein called keratin, but did you know that the body also uses it in fingernails? Here are some of the more weird and wonderful facts you may have missed about your fog hat.

Hair Facts

The average head has some 100,000 strands of hair on it.

A blonde usually has many more strands on their head than those with red or dark locks.

Everyone loses at least 40 to 100 strands of hair a day.

Hair has two distinct structures: the follicle that sits beneath the skin and the shaft that extends above the skin surface.

A single hair has a thickness of 0.02mm–0.04mm.

It would take a force equivalent to 60kg to tear a strand of hair, which is equivalent to a strand of iron.

We are born with all our hair follicles which are programmed to grow hair.

Baldness can be passed down through either the paternal or maternal line.

Hair and Hairstyling Records

Wherever there is a record to be broken you can be sure there is a queue of mentalists keen to do so. Here is our list of those who inexplicably went the extra mile for their entry in *The Guinness Book of World Records*.

World's Longest Hair

Vietnam's Tran Van Hay holds the current record for having the world's longest hair. At the time of his death aged 79, some estimates put the length of his unwashed locks at 6.8m. Hay had begun to let his hair grow more than fifty years previously, because – he claimed – he often got sick after having a haircut. During the day Hay balanced his mighty locks – which weighed several pounds – on his head like a basket, and protected them with a scarf. Unfortunately this rendered him housebound as he was banned from taking the local motorcycle taxis because he could not wear a helmet. His wife, Nguyen Thi Hoa, said of the great man, 'He lived a simple life as a herbalist, but his hair could complicate things.' Something of an understatement.

Most Scissors Used in a Haircut

On 11 March 2002, America's Bruce Choy successfully styled hair using a record-breaking eight pairs of scissors simultaneously in one hand. Choy invented his 'Flyingshears' technique after seeing guitarist Stanley Jordan playing two guitars at once. Choy explained, 'I thought, I've been cutting hair for twenty years and my left hand is always helping the right but I started to train the other hand ... they became like one hand, and I can be perfect.' Choy, who's also known by some wags as 'Edward Scissorhands', beat the previous record of seven scissors, held by Israel's Danny Bar-Gil.

Largest Collection of Celebrity Hair

There's nothing creepy about hair enthusiast John Reznikoff of Connecticut, USA, who has dedicated his life to accumulating a collection of human hair from some 115 celebrities. His bizarre collection includes historical political figures of note such as Abraham Lincoln, Napoleon, John F. Kennedy and King Charles I, as well as follicles of the famous from the world of entertainment like Marilyn Monroe, Elvis Presley and Charles Dickens. He even has a lock of Albert Einstein's trademark grey frizz. His collection of famous locks is insured for a cool $1 million.

Largest Wig

Everyone loves a full head of hair but for those who find themselves thinning on top, there is always a wig. Not surprisingly, people have been drawn to make these creations bigger and better. The largest wig on record was made from human hair. It was created by Bergmann of Fifth Avenue, New York in 1975. This monster syrup measured a staggering 4.57m (15ft) in length. Interestingly, unlike the people who wear them, the record books don't make much distinction around the composition of these distracting monstrosities. They can be made from real human hair or from animal hair – commonly from horses and goats – or more recently, from synthetic materials.

Most Valuable Hair

We'd all like to leave something for our kids when we die, but very few of us think of leaving our hair. The most valuable hair clippings ever sold at auction were some dark black curls from the head of the king of rock 'n' roll himself, Elvis Presley. The off cuts were sold by his personal barber, Homer 'Gill' Gilleland, for $115,120 (£72,791), as part of an online auction of memorabilia on 15 November 2002. The King's rockabilly rug went to an anonymous bidder.

Most Valuable Hair on a Living Person

Professional sportsman Troy Polamalu holds the dubious honour of having the world's most expensive hair. The well-known American football player plays in defence for the Pittsburgh Steelers, and the long, black mane which protrudes from the back of his helmet has become a touchstone for fans of the team. So recognisable are Polamalu's long black curls, that he has an endorsement contract with Head & Shoulders shampoo. In August 2010, the shampoo's owners Proctor & Gamble paid to insure the player's hair for $1 million, with Lloyd's of London.

Strongest Hair

The world's strongest hair probably belongs to 44-year-old He Jian Ma from China's Hunan province. In 2009 he used a special steel ring woven into his rug to pull a bus weighing over 8 tonnes across an eye-watering distance of 30m. The feat beat Jian Ma's previous record for hair pulling in which he dragged a 2-tonne car over 15m.

Most Heads Shaved

It might seem an easy task to complete, but the most heads shaved in four hours is a breathtaking 662. The feat was achieved by a team of five hairstylists from Sears Hair Studio at Notre Dame College in Ontario on 8 April 2006. History does not record who had to clean up the salon afterwards.

Tallest Mohawk

The hard rocking honour of having the world's tallest Mohawk is held by Eric Hahn, the guitarist of punk band The Filthy Few. On 14 November 2008, Hahn had the sides of his head shaved in the presence of a Guinness World Record adjudicator and the record-breaking Hawk was raised. The measurement came to 68.58cm, or 27in, which beat the previous record of 24in.

Fastest Haircut and Most Haircuts Completed

Ivan Zoot is the Usain Bolt of barbering and holder of not one, but three, Guinness World Records for haircutting. A professional barber from Austin, Texas, Zoot set the records during a fundraising event for the charity Children with Hair Loss. In a single exhausting session he broke the record for the fastest single haircut (a layered bob performed in fifty-five seconds), the most professional haircuts in one hour (thirty-four) and the most haircuts in twenty-four hours (340). To achieve the latter, he cut hair from 4 p.m. on a Friday, until 4 p.m. the next day, cutting non-stop (except for seven quick bathroom breaks of five minutes or less). During this time, he averaged one haircut every 4.23 minutes.

Longest Hair Extensions

The world longest hair extensions are owned by a Kiwi, Alastair Galpinhas, who had 6.68m of synthetic hair woven into his hairline. The extensions were added at the Garden of Eve hair salon in St Heliers, New Zealand, over a period of four hours. It is worth noting that professional record nutter Galpinhas is also the holder of some seventy-five other world records, including having the most snails on a human face (eight in ten seconds), the most rubber-bands stretched over a face (sixty-two in one minute) and the most stamps licked in one minute (fifty-seven).

Longest Time Hanging by your Hair

Most of us like to keep our 'dos in shape, but Sri Lankan-born Suthakaran Sivagnanathurai has such strong tresses that he was able to set a new world record in Queensland, Australia. He spent twenty-three minutes dangling by his hair more than a metre off the ground. He later said, 'My hair is strong because I usually use natural oil.' He went on to say that he had overcome the pain of the process by meditating.

Highest Hairstyle

The world's highest hairstyle was constructed on the 21 June 2009 at the Frisör salon in Wels, Austria. The towering top piece was fashioned by several hairstylists working together using real (and some fake) hair in the gobsmacking construction. When they finished, it measured in at a lofty 2.66m (8.73ft). It's not known if anyone has actually worn the wig.

Endurance Hairdressing

While there are multiple feats of endurance hairdressing in the record books, Patrick Lomantini can still lay claim to the longest period of continuous hairdressing undertaken. He managed to climb his own personal Everest of 227 cuts during a non-stop seventy-two-hour session, to set a Guinness World Record for endurance haircutting. The attempt took place at Lomantini's salon in Wichita, Kansas, during which Lomantini relied on a twelve-person support team to sweep the floor of the salon, as well as providing food and drinks day and night. He also kept two massage therapists on site who gave him a well-deserved rubdown every three hours.

Quotes about Hair

It's not just teenagers on the pull, rock stars and balding men who are obsessed by their hair. For most of us it's something that is constantly on our mind and often in our hands. Here's what the great and the good have to say about it.

A good man might be hard to find, but a good hairdresser is next to impossible.

Unknown

There's many a man has more hair than wit.

William Shakespeare

Gray hair is God's graffiti.

Bill Cosby

I don't consider myself bald, I'm just taller than my hair.

Lucius Annaeus Seneca

There are times when I flick through magazines and think I'm in danger of becoming a prisoner of my own hair.

Brian May

✂---

Thy boist'rous locks, no worthy match
For valour to assail, nor by the sword
But by the barber's razor best subdued.

John Milton

✂---

Long hair is an unpardonable offence which should be punishable by death.

Steven Morrissey

✂---

The hair is real – it's the head that's a fake.

Steve Allen

✂---

Babies haven't any hair:
Old men's heads are just as bare;
From the cradle to the grave
Lies a haircut and a shave.

Samuel Goodman Hoffenstein

✂---

For me the working of hair is architecture with a human element.

Vidal Sassoon

✂--

Inflation is when you pay fifteen dollars for the ten-dollar haircut you used to get for five dollars when you had hair.

Sam Ewing

✂--

Beckham? His wife can't sing and his barber can't cut hair.

Brian Clough

✂--

Hair is vitally personal to children. They weep vigorously when it is cut for the first time; no matter how it grows, bushy, straight or curly, they feel they are being shorn of a part of their personality.

Charlie Chaplin

✂--

You're only as good as your last haircut.

Fran Lebowitz

✂--

Beauty isn't worth thinking about; what's important is your mind. You don't want a fifty-dollar haircut on a fifty-cent head.

Garrison Keillor

✂---

Never ask a barber if you need a haircut.

Cowboy proverb

✂---

Some of the worst mistakes in my life were haircuts.

Jim Morrison

✂---

All things change except barbers, the ways of barbers, and the surroundings of barbers. These never change.

Mark Twain

✂---

We're all born bald, baby.

Telly Savalas

✂---

Ridiculous Names for Hair Salons

When it comes to the naming of their place of business, hairdressers lead the field in falling back on horrendous puns. Hairdressing is a competitive business and ever since the first ready wit felt that calling their salon 'A cut above the rest' might in some way help to attract trade, snippers the world over have competed to choose the most ridiculous and tenuous puns to describe the work they do inside. Here is a small section of the worst.

The Best Little Hairhouse
Beyond the Fringe
British Hairways

Cliptomania
Clip Teasers
Comb One, Comb All
Combing Attractions
Con Hair
Crops and Bobbers
Curl up and Dye
Cut-n-edge

Director's Cut
Dye Hard
To Dye For

From Hair to Eternity

Grateful Head

Hair & Now
Hair & There
Hair-After
Hair Apparent
Hair Force
Hairatage
The Hair Port
The Hairtaker
Hair Today (Gone Tomorrow)
Hairway to Heaven
Headmasters
Headonizm
His and Hairs
The Head Shed

Julius Scissor

Killin Kutz

The Locks Smith
Loose Ends
Lunatic Fringe

The Mane Attraction
Millionhairs

Shear Genius
Shear-n-dipity
Sunny and Shear

Talking Heads

Wave Lengths

THE WORLD OF HAIRSTYLES

If you enjoyed this book, you may also be interested in…

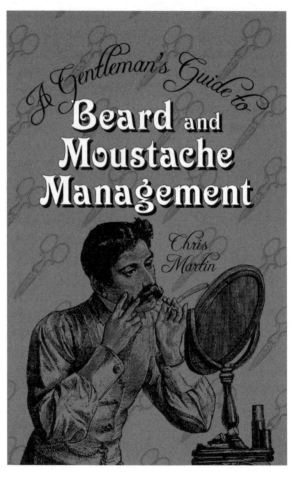

978 0 7524 5975 2

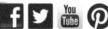